Secrets About the HCG Diet!

- Treatment Guide
- Controversy
- Benefits
- Risks
- Side Effects
- Contraindications

Look great!
Feel great!
Lose weight!
Have better sex!

Y.L. Wright, M.A.

Book Five in the Series,
"Bioidentical Hormones."

MEDICAL DISCLAIMER:

The following text is for general information only. It contains the opinions and ideas of the author. Careful attention has been paid to insure the accuracy of the information, but the author and the publisher cannot assume responsibility for the validity or consequences of its use. The intention of this book is to provide helpful information. This information is not intended to diagnose or treat any disease. This book is sold with the understanding that the author and publisher are not rendering medical, health, or any other professional services. See your medical or health professional concerning any health concerns or before following any suggestions made in this book or drawing inferences from it. The author and publisher specifically disclaim all responsibility for any liability, loss, or risk incurred as a direct or indirect consequence of using this book's contents. Any use of the information found in this book is the sole responsibility of the reader. Any dietary, nutrient, hormone, and medication suggestions found in this book are to be followed only under the supervision of a medical doctor or other endocrine specialist. Any reference to particular companies or supplements is only for the benefit of the reader. The author receives no compensation from endorsement of any product.

ACKNOWLEDGMENTS:

Back cover picture courtesy of Joe Swartz, MD. Thanks also to Dr. Swartz for editing this manuscript for medical accuracy.

FDA DISCLAIMER:

HCG has not been demonstrated to be an effective adjunctive therapy in the treatment of obesity. There is no substantial evidence that it increases weight loss beyond that resulting from caloric restriction, that it causes a more attractive or normal distribution of fat, or that it decreases the hunger or discomfort associated with calorie-restricted diets.

Table of Contents

Introduction

HCG IS ONE OF THE BIOIDENTICAL HORMONES that can help us to normalize the hormone imbalances that result from dieting and aging. Although hCG is not a hormone involved in the hormonal imbalance caused by aging and dieting, the use of hCG (human Chorionic Gonadotropin) may be an effective aid to lose unwanted fat and to assist you in getting your hormones balanced.

Increasing numbers of people have been using hCG coupled with a low-calorie diet to lose weight. They are reporting weight loss without a loss of energy. They say that they feel an increase in well-being and a renewed sense of vitality.

The big problem with hCG is that it's hard to find accurate information about it. Everyone is trying to make money off of it. When you try to find information about hCG on the internet, you will be referred to the hCG preparation that they are trying to sell. These people have a vested interest in biasing you toward their particular product.

Many books are also biased. Instead of references to scientific studies, you may be referred to their website selling their hCG product.

I am only interested in your health. I have no interest in selling you an hCG product. The purpose of this book is to present the facts about weight loss, hormonal balance, and hCG in an unbiased manner.

We will look at the pros AND the cons of hCG dieting. You should know what you're getting into before you decide to use this controversial fat-loss method. Read this book and learn the facts about hCG--the benefits, the warnings, the off-label usage, the contradictions, and the contraindications.

HCG is a hormone that is normally produced in pregnancy. How can taking a pregnancy hormone help both non-pregnant women and men to lose weight and keep it off?

Let's find out how it works. What's the scoop? Is it dangerous? Does it keep the weight off? How is it taken to work most effectively? What are the specifics of the hCG diet protocol? What are the side effects? How can I do the diet safely? What else do I need to know to take the weight off and keep it off? These are all questions that will be answered in this book, backed up by relevant research.

This book is the fifth book in my series, "Bioidentical Hormones." My mission in writing these books is to bring you the latest scientific information gleaned from hundreds of lectures given by anti-aging physicians and supported by the research presented in scientific journals.

Read the other books in the "Bioidentical Hormones" series by Y.L. Wright, M.A.:

(1) Secrets about Bioidentical Hormones to Lose Fat and Prevent Cancer, Heart Disease, Menopause, and Andropause by Optimizing Adrenals, Thyroid, Estrogen, Progesterone, Testosterone, and Growth Hormone!

(2) Bioidentical Hormones Made Easy!

(3) Secrets About Growth Hormone to Build Muscle, Increase Bone Density, and Burn Body Fat!

(4) Fat Loss Secrets that Really Work! Balance Your Hormones: Insulin, Estrogen, Progesterone, Testosterone, Thyroid, Cortisol, and DHEA!

All of my books can be purchased in either print or downloadable versions at:
http://www.lulu.com/spotlight/treewise

1. What is HCG?

HCG, HUMAN CHORIONIC GONADOTROPIN, is a hormone produced in pregnancy by the placenta.

- *"Chorionic" means the placenta makes it.* It is not a woman that makes it. It is not a man that makes it. The placenta makes it.

- *"Gonadotropin" means that it will stimulate the gonads,* the sex organs, in both men and women. In pregnancy, hCG stimulates the production of progesterone, allowing the uterus to sustain a growing fetus. In men, it acts like LH (luteinizing hormone), to increase testosterone production.

- *HCG controls metabolic functions* during pregnancy. It has been hypothesized that the hCG that is produced during pregnancy acts on the hypothalamus in the brain. The hypothalamus will then signal the mother's fat stores to nourish the fetus if the woman is not eating enough during pregnancy. The hCG that is produced by the placenta will provide nutrition for the baby by obtaining calories from the mother's fat reserves, sparing the mother's muscle mass.

- *HCG controls appetite.* HCG increases leptin.[1] Leptin's role in the body is to produce feelings of satiety after meals.

- *HCG is also believed to override the mother's immune system* to allow her to carry a baby that is different from herself without rejecting it as non-self.[2] [3]

- *HCG is what is detected in home pregnancy tests.* A positive pregnancy test shows hCG in the urine.

- ***The hCG that is used in medicine is extracted from the urine of pregnant women.*** In the later stages of pregnancy, the placenta can make up to a million units a day. It is tested in the lab for potency and sterilization.

- ***In non-pregnant people, hCG increases metabolism to a rate similar to a pregnant female.***[4] HCG produces the release of stored fat calories. The hCG acts on the hypothalamus to secrete a fat-mobilizing substance that stops fat formation (lipogenesis).[5]

- ***HCG is used in weight loss programs.*** It facilitates weight loss by accessing the reserves of stored fat to be burned as energy, just as it does in pregnancy. Releasing these fat stores can provide up to 2000-3000 calories per day depending on the size of the patient. These calories can be used for energy, preventing the hunger and fatigue that are typical with other low-calorie diets.

- ***HCG works by raising the metabolism.*** When given to men, their testosterone levels go up, which causes metabolism to increase.

- ***When men have hypogonadism, or low testosterone, hCG is one way of bringing their testosterone levels back up.*** HCG stimulates the testes to produce more testosterone naturally. Therefore, there is no atrophy of the pituitary-testosterone system and no testicular atrophy. Young men in their 20's and 30's often have very low testosterone levels when they are under a lot of stress. These men may benefit from an improved diet, decreased stress, and increased zinc. HCG is a natural substance that may raise testosterone without lowering sperm count, if they want to reproduce.[6] HCG will increase testosterone levels and support increased spermatogenesis. Testosterone therapy is another option that may be used if they do not care about keeping their sperm count up. Testosterone may be used temporarily until they can build their own production back up by improving lifestyle.

- *In women, hCG is used to treat infertility* by stimulating ovulation and allowing for the final maturation of eggs.[7]

- *Injection of hCG produces a sense of well-being. Many people do not want to stop taking it after the treatment period ends.* It acts in the hypothalamus to produce satiety and to increase a sense of well-being.[8] After the hCG is administered, it accumulates in the hypothalamic region.[9] The beta-endorphin content in the hCG molecule causes opioid modulation of the hypothalamus, creating a good mood during treatment.[10]

Let's look next at how hCG has been used successfully to help people lose weight.

2. HCG in a Program to Lose Fat

MOST DIETS WITH SEVERE CALORIC RESTRICTION have the great disadvantage of the loss of lean muscle along with the fat loss. The loss of lean muscle mass slows metabolism, encouraging weight gain. It becomes a vicious cycle of weight lost and impaired metabolism with each dieting attempt.

> ### Diets that specifically cause muscle loss:
> * Starvation and ketosis dieting.
> * Eating less than 800 calories a day (without hCG).
> * Long-term appetite suppressants.
> * Diets that recommend eating less than three meals a day.

As lean muscle is lost, metabolism drops more and more. It becomes a vicious cycle of losing weight and rapidly regaining it, because metabolism is impaired. The more you diet, the more difficult it becomes to lose the weight.

There are three types of fat:

1) **Structural fat** protects the organs, bones, coronary arteries, and keeps the skin tight.

2) **Normal fat** is used for muscular activity and maintenance of body temperature. It is found all over the body. Structural and normal types of fat do not cause obesity.

3) **Abnormal fat** is the accumulation of fat on the belly, hips, thighs, and arms. It is not readily available to the body in a nutritional emergency. Abnormal fat doesn't burn off easily with regular dieting.

During starvation or very-low-calorie diets, the first fat to be used is the normal fat, then the structural fat, then finally the abnormal fat. The skin wrinkles. The fat needed to protect the organs and bones decreases, while the excess fat on belly, hips, thighs, and upper arms remains. Weakness, hunger, depression, and frustration lead to abandonment of the diet.

Dr. Simeons found that hCG helped his patients to lose fat without losing their lean muscle. Fifty-seven years ago, Dr. A.T. Simeons decided to try using hCG supplementation in non-pregnant women and males on a low calorie diet to see if it would increase their metabolism like it does in pregnant women.[11] [12]

He noticed that the metabolism of obese people is different from that of normal people, and that their fat is more resistant to dieting. Simeons hypothesized that obesity originates in the hypothalamus and is due to a neuropeptide concentration imbalance. This imbalance causes people to accumulate fat. He wanted to see if hCG could over-ride this imbalance and allow obese patients to lose unhealthy fat.

His patients lost about a pound a day. They lost fat, not lean muscle. They lost the abnormal fat, the belly fat, not the normal or structural fat. They lost inches around the belly, hips, and thighs. Their skin remained tight. They did not experience the problems associated with very low calorie diets. While following his hCG diet, his patients did not experience the hunger, weakness, and irritability associated with low calorie diets without hCG. They had no headaches, hunger, cravings, weakness, or irritability. He reported that the hCG had no undesirable side effects.

Simeons' diet concepts included elimination of simple sugars, trans fats, and chemically processed food and drink. His patients stayed at his clinic where they ate mostly protein, fruits, and vegetables and drank a minimum of eight 8-ounce glasses of water each day. He injected them with 150-200 IU's of hCG once a day for a 21-day or 42-day cycle while placing them on a diet of 500 calories a day for three or six weeks.

Simeons found that it was very important to stop the hCG after a three-week or six-week period because patients developed a tolerance to it. The three-week period is used for those who don't have as much weight to lose and are doing it more for esthetics rather than to lose a large amount of weight. Then after a period of time, they could do another cycle if they still needed to lose more weight. After a period of time, the cycle may be repeated again if more fat loss is desired. Cycling the HCG in exactly this way has proven to be the most successful way to lose the unwanted fat and keep it off. A longer break is taken between the second and third cycle than between the first and second cycle.

Over the years since Dr. Simeons developed the hCG protocol, tens of thousands of people have used some version of Simeons' hCG diet and have lost weight quickly, safely, and kept it off. Daniel Belluscio, M.D. has treated over 6000 patients using Simeons' protocol with no complications. He combines hCG with liposuction to get the best results.[13]

Many people are reporting amazing results using hCG to lose weight. They are able to get down to previously unattainable weights, even though they used roller-coasting dieting methods for most of their lives. Their muscle mass goes up, so they look a lot better, and their metabolism is improved.

Proponents say that HCG targets the abnormal fat and spares lean muscle. Proponents of hCG therapy claim that when using hCG, the abnormal fat is the first to go. HCG works in both men and women by targeting abnormal fat while on a very low calorie diet. HCG will not cause weight loss unless it is combined with caloric restriction. Proponents say that hCG is beneficial in a weight loss program because:

- It spares lean muscle.
- It protects the structural fat.
- It redistributes fat.
- It decreases cravings for sweets.
- It decreases appetite.
- It increases libido.
- It maintains weight loss even after returning to regular calorie intake.
- It ends yo-yo dieting frustration.
- It is ideal for women in menopause whose hormone levels are declining or imbalanced.

3. This is How HCG Works its Magic

PROPONENTS CLAIM THAT HCG SHRINKS YOUR FAT CELLS. HCG is believed to work by causing the hypothalamus (the master gland in the brain) to target and mobilize stored nutrients within the fat cells. It mobilizes these stored nutrients by shrinking and draining the contents of the fat cells.

Proponents also say that HCG gives you energy while you diet. In a non-pregnant person, these nutrients are released into the bloodstream to be used as energy or eliminated. (In pregnant women, these nutrients would go to the fetus.) Up to 2000 calories may be released in a day, decreasing hunger and increasing energy and metabolism. If the body doesn't use all the calories, it eliminates them. Because the nutrients can be used for energy, you don't feel hungry or tired, as you do on other diets.

HCG elevates sex hormone levels, which increases metabolism. Very-low-calorie diets without hCG result in decreases in the levels of these important hormones, thus lowering metabolism.

HCG causes rapid weight loss. Weight loss clinics that use hCG claim that post-menopausal women and women who have had a hysterectomy lose about 25 pounds in 40 days. Women of child-bearing age lose more weight, about 25-35 pounds, due to higher metabolic and hormonal levels.

Men have higher metabolic rates than women because of increased testosterone production. The weight-loss clinics say that men will lose about a pound a day, or 30-45 pounds in 40 days.

Both sexes report loss of inches. They drop to smaller sizes in their clothing and maintain it over the long run.

4.   **Treatment Modalities**

THE MOST EFFECTIVE WAY TO TAKE HCG is in the injectable form available only by prescription from a physician. The injections can be taken subcutaneously or intramuscularly. Studies have shown that either way works just about as well for weight loss, but intra-muscular provides better bio-availability.[14] For fifty years, Dr. Simeons in Great Britain was using intramuscular injections. This is the source of most of the data that we have about hCG.

Today most people use subcutaneous injections because it is easier and less painful. Your doctor can teach you how to inject it yourself.   One of the downsides with the injectable forms is that they must be kept cold, which is difficult when you are traveling. One upside is that using a needle to inject the hormone every day sets a serious tone to the protocol.   The process of injecting this potent hormone reminds the patient of how important it is to follow the structure of the protocol exactly. The injection method also insures adequate absorption of the hCG in order to get the best results.

Other forms of hCG are not as effective. Recently, compounding pharmacies have been offering other forms.

Sublingual (under the tongue), intranasal, and transdermal (through the skin) must be given at twice the subcutaneous dosage. Transdermal forms don't have to be kept cold, but have not proven to be as effective as the injectable forms.

Sublingual hCG is not reliable. When using sublingual administration, you will not get a positive serum pregnancy test, which suggests that this form doesn't deliver adequate levels of hCG. You must hold it under your tongue for a certain period of time, and most people swallow a significant amount, which inactivates it. Sublingual is not nearly as reliable as injectable in terms of bringing blood levels of hCG high enough to get the response that you need.

Homeopathic hCG is the least effective choice. Homeopathic hCG preparations may be effective for some people. You can try it and see. These are diluted concentrations of hCG. The dilutions vary. Because they are not regulated, some may not even have any hCG at all. But even if they are somewhat effective, homeopathic alternatives are not the big guns. Most people don't get the results that they would if they used hCG as prescribed by a physician.

Although some forms of hCG are now available without a physician's prescription, read on before you consider going it on your own. Once you get started on the program with a doctor, you don't have to go in and see your doctor very often unless you are going in weekly to get a MIC injection, which I will explain in a minute. You can call your doctor to report your results as you go along.

There are many things that can go wrong on this protocol, especially when done incorrectly. Your health is your only real wealth, so my advice is to protect yourself by only undergoing the protocol under the supervision of a knowledgeable health-care professional with a long history of using the hCG protocol.[15] Undergoing severe calorie restriction may result in serious health complications, whether done with or without hCG.[16]

Before using the HCG protocol, use the weight-loss methods that have been proven to work.

These methods are described in detail in Book Four of the "Bioidentical Hormone" series, <u>Fat Loss Secrets that Really Work! Balance Your Hormones: Insulin, Estrogen, Progesterone, Testosterone, Thyroid, Cortisol, and DHEA!</u>[17]

5. Find a Physician Who Prescribes HCG for Weight Loss

FIND A DOCTOR WHO IS KNOWLEDGEABLE in the use of hCG to help people lose weight. If you are unable to find a doctor in your area who is willing to treat you with hCG for weight loss, you may be able to find one who will treat you with hCG by searching through the physicians associated with the American Academy of Anti-Aging Medicine (A4M)[18] or American College for Advancement in Medicine (ACAM).[19] These anti-aging and functional medicine doctors are practicing state-of-the-art medicine, the medicine conservative physicians will be practicing in forty years.

American Academy of Anti-Aging Medicine (A4M)
888-997-0112   http://www.worldhealth.net/

American College for Advancement in Medicine (ACAM)
800-532-3688   http://www.acamnet.org

When you go to an M.D. or D.O. who prescribes hCG, you will get a consultation, labs, history, and physical. Labs recommended are CBC, Chem panel, and TSH/T3/T4. Women will need estradiol labs. Pre-menopausal women also need to get an hCG test to make sure that they are not pregnant. Men will need free and total testosterone labs. If you want to move into more hormone supplementation, you will need to get a more comprehensive hormone profile.

Your doctor will take your history and give you a physical. It is especially important to test estrogen metabolism to screen for cancer risk. An effective diet plan should be carefully reviewed with the patient for use during the injection protocol. The patient must be informed of off-label use.

It is the physician's responsibility before administering the hCG protocol to first, "Do no harm." Each patient should receive a thorough patient examination and a medical history should be taken. Ample follow-up should be provided during the protocol. An effective diet plan should be carefully reviewed with the patient for use during the injection protocol. The patient must be informed of off-label use. The FDA and the courts allow the use of hCG in an off-label way. But it must be documented as informed consent in the patient's chart.

Your doctor should monitor your hormone levels and metabolism and keep them in the proper range. Women using supplemental estradiol and progesterone before beginning hCG may need to cut down on their replacement doses, as hCG will raise these hormone levels.[20] [21] [22]

As the weight is lost, estrogen may decrease. Less fat means less aromatization and estrogen in post-menopausal women. Estrogen levels fall as fat decreases.

6. A Guide to Doing the HCG Protocol

CLEAN UP YOUR DIET before you start. At least two weeks before beginning the hCG diet, eliminate processed foods, sweets, fried foods, high-fructose corn syrup, alcohol, and artificial sweeteners. Eat organic foods. You need to get used to eating this way because it will make the diet more effective. Your body needs time to adjust to eating better foods and to eliminate the toxicity caused by poor eating habits.

The hCG weight loss protocol lasts for 4-6 weeks taking the hCG. Your doctor will prescribe the hCG for 40 days. People who don't need to lose as much weight may see the results they are seeking in as little as 21 days. Walk and follow the 500 calorie a day diet protocol. Scrupulously follow your doctor's instructions. The calorie restriction must be followed if you want to get the results. You will need to take supplements, and follow the diet protocol and food guide.

Nutrition is extremely important. Because of the calorie restriction, nutrients are also being restricted. So it is important to supplement with plenty of nutrients needed for good health. You should take multi vitamins and minerals, Co-Q10, probiotics, Omega 3's, B-complex, and anti-oxidants. MIC injections (methionine, inositol, choline, vitamin B-12, and chromium) may be taken weekly or monthly. These nutrients help to break down and metabolize fats and carbohydrates, and aid in digestion, absorption, protein synthesis, insulin sensitivity, and maintenance of proper blood sugar levels.

During the next 4-6 weeks, men may continue to use the hCG to keep their testosterone levels up. But women should take 4-6 weeks off from the hCG to let the body stabilize. Women's estrogen and progesterone may drop during this time, so they may want to add these hormones. Please see books one and two in the "Bioidentical Hormone" series for specific information about using supplemental estrogen and progesterone.[23][24] After the 4-6 weeks off of the hCG, if a woman needs to lose more weight, she can do another hCG round of 4-6 weeks.

7. The Four Phases of the hCG Protocol

THE FOUR PHASES OF THE HCG PROTOCOL
ARE:
    (1) Loading.
    (2) Transformation.
    (3) Stabilization.
    (4) Maintenance.

Phase 1, loading, insures that you will not gain the weight back. You should prepare for the hCG injections by cleansing. Cleanse to detoxify for seven to thirty days. Use herbs that detox the intestines. Coffee enemas are good to do at this time to help eliminate the fat-soluble toxins that are being released into the blood stream from the fat stores. Load up on carbs for the last week before beginning Phase 2 to build up your normal fat reserves that may have been depleted during other diets. Drink at least a half gallon of water a day and work up to a gallon of water every day. Continue drinking lots of water for the rest of your life.

Phase 2, transformation, lasts between 3-6 weeks. You will lose unwanted abnormal fat deposits. This is when you begin to inject the hCG. Energy should be high and hunger and appetite low as you lose around a pound a day.

The injections take three days to begin working, so during the first two days of the hCG injections, you may still eat as much as you want. Continue loading up on carbs. Eat grains like brown rice, sweet potatoes, oatmeal, and so forth for the first two days. This increases your fat stores to prepare you for the strict diet.

On the third day you will eat begin to eat only 500 calories a day divided into three meals: Some protocols recommend a protein, a fruit, and a vegetable at every meal. The protein should be varied at each meal and changed from day to day to avoid becoming allergic to any one protein.

On the hCG diet, you are not allowed to eat and drink foods which contain fats/oil. You may not use oil on your skin. The diet calls for:

- 100 grams (4 oz) of protein split into 2 servings per day, broiled or grilled.
- Two servings of vegetables a day.
- Two servings of fruit per day (apple, orange, ½ grapefruit, handful of strawberries).
- One Melba toast or bread stick daily.
- Drink ½ to one gallon of water a day and coffee or tea with no sugar.
- Although not recommended, if you exercise strenuously, you may eat five meals a day.

During the last three days of the transformation diet you will stop taking the hCG, but continue on the 500-calorie diet. After the three days, it is OK to eat normally, because then all the hCG will have been eliminated. It is important not to eat normally until all the hCG is eliminated, because weight is gained easily when there is still hCG in the system.

On the 40th day, do another cleanse. Again, detoxify for seven days. Take herbs that detox the intestines. Coffee enemas are an invaluable aid to eliminating the fat-soluble toxicity that is being released into the blood stream. You don't want those toxins to be re-absorbed into the tissues.

Phase 3, stabilization, begins on day 43. This phase resets the body weight set point permanently. For the first three weeks, you will increase calories to 800-1000 daily over three meals a day, or five meals a day if you exercise strenuously. You are resetting your metabolism higher, hunger lower, and teaching your hypothalamus not to store fat in abnormal fat reserves.

During this phase, eat slowly and stop eating when full. Weigh yourself every day. Increase exercise. You may begin resistance training. You may eat proteins, fruits, or vegetables, but no starchy carbohydrates or sugars.

For the next three weeks on the stabilization phase, you will increase your calories to 1250-1500 starting the 57th day by adding two or three more meals a day. You may eat more low-glycemic and low-fat foods. You are not eating any starchy carbs, but you are eating a little more protein and a little more fruit. Increase the number of meals to 5 or 6 a day. Now you can begin doing more resistance exercises. If exercising a lot, you may eat 6 or 7 meals daily. This is often the time when you lose more inches and fat, even though you are not taking hCG.

Trouble-shooting "steak day." If you gain more than 2 pounds in a day, skip all food until 6 pm, drink at least a gallon of water and teas, and in the evening eat a big steak (grass-fed organic, grilled, no salt) and a large organic raw tomato or large raw apple.

Phase 4, maintenance, lasts the rest of your life. The new weight set-point must be maintained. It is important to eat small amounts of food to satisfy hunger. Sugars and starches are slowly re-introduced. Food choices and portion sizes are increased.

You will eat just enough calories to maintain the weight loss. You find this number of calories by multiplying your goal weight by 13. A female who has hit her goal weight of 140 pounds would multiply 140 by 13. That would be 1820 calories a day to maintain that weight of 140 pounds.

If you follow the maintenance phase, you will keep the weight off. If you start to gain weight, you must increase your exercise and/or drop your calories. You will regain the weight if you go back to eating fast foods, eating high-glycemic loads, restaurant food, trans fats, high fructose corn syrup, sugar, artificial sweeteners, foods with hormones and antibiotics, preservatives, and junk food. It helps to weigh yourself to keep focused. Better yet, look in the mirror.

Bioidentical hormones may be used during or after the hCG protocol. Metabolism will increase when the hormones are balanced and optimized. Belly fat will reduce and age-related diseases associated with weight gain will be prevented. Optimum hormone levels will increase energy and increase lean muscle mass.

8. Tips to Keep the Fat Off!

- ***A****VOID FAST FOODS.*
- Keep eating a low glycemic, high protein diet.
- Avoid more than one starch daily.
- Limit refined sugar, preservatives.
- Avoid food additives. MSG, sugar, hydrogenated fats, preservatives, food coloring, and all chemicals.
- Drink lots of water.
- Eat only organic food and organic tea.
- Exercise often (at least three times per week for 20-30 minutes).
- If cortisol is elevated, it will increase appetite and cravings for sweets. The stress will put fat in undesirable locations. Stress will decrease the other hormones that drop with age. Take adaptogens to normalize cortisol levels. These include ashwaganda (taken in the afternoon or evening), holy basil (evening), ginseng, rhodiola, and others.[25]
- DHEA studies show that taking DHEA may reduce post-diet obesity. It targets fat loss in the abdomen. In weight loss, DHEA stimulates enzymes in the liver to burn fat.
- Adequate thyroid hormone is necessary to maintain higher metabolic rates and keep the fat off.[26]
- Bioidentical Sex Hormone Replacement Therapy (BHRT). When you go off hCG, begin BHRT as needed. BHRT increases metabolism by optimizing and balancing hormones.[27]
- Optimize Growth Hormone. Optimal GH levels are important to keep losing fat, maintain muscle, and lose weight in the long run. It helps to maintain higher IGF-1 levels which reduce body fat and prevent the age-related diseases associated with weight gain. Be sure to read my book about Growth Hormone,[28] as there are very serious risks involved when using supplemental Human Growth Hormone and GH stimulators.
- Supplement with testosterone if low. Low testosterone in both men and women may contribute to low energy, fatigue, decreased muscle mass, and fat storage. Adding testosterone will stimulate fat-burning. If women are adding supplemental estrogen, but their testosterone is low, the estrogen may facilitate fat storage.

9.   Health May Improve After Using HCG

PREVIOUSLY DIABETIC PATIENTS *may not need to restart their meds or may lower their medications after finishing the protocol,* because they may no longer require the meds to control their blood sugar. A 6-week course of hCG has proven to be one of the most effective treatments to improve the health of a type-2 diabetic.[29] Never stop diabetic medication except under the supervision of your physician.

Some physicians may stop prescribing thyroid medication while on the diet because of the structural similarity between hCG and TSH. Others may keep thyroid meds the same because they haven't seen clinical change in thyroid symptoms or change in thyroid labs during the diet.

HCG has a long history of safety. If problems occur, it is usually because of other diseases present—diabetes, heart disease, etc. HCG has been used for decades [30] [31] [32] in both men and women in much greater dosages than those used for weight management without many problems. When compared to other weight loss methods, the hCG protocol compares favorably in terms of risk and possibility of harm. The gonadal stimulation that occurs with the use of hCG does not appear to place the patient at any greater risk, except for ovarian hyperstimulation syndrome. Lower doses reduce this risk.[33] It boosts feelings of well-being.

HCG has been shown to reduce the risk of an established tumor getting worse. It reduces the chances of developing breast or ovarian cancer. The news is all good in terms of breast cancer risk.[34] [35]

Chronic pain may disappear while on the hCG protocol. Many patients who have chronic pain and do the hCG protocol report complete remission of their pain without taking their pain medication. But the pain returns when they discontinue the hGH. They are happy with the weight loss, but not with the return of their pain and other inflammatory conditions. In fact, hCG has been used in Europe for years to treat inflammation.[36]

10. The Benefits of HCG for Weight Loss

- **WEIGHT LOSS IS TARGETED.** Fat is lost, not muscle. Structural fat is protected. Problem fat (belly, buttocks, and thighs) is targeted.
- Weight loss within a six-week period is rapid relative to other weight-loss methods.
- It increases metabolism.
- It decreases cravings and appetite.
- It increases libido in both men and women.
- It ends roller-coaster dieting.
- It helps to remove those last difficult 10-20 pounds impossible to lose with other weight-loss methods
- It may be used to lose a large amount of weight or for just 10-20 lbs.
- It helps to balance hormone levels in aging.
- It is well-tolerated by most people when done properly.
- There is usually mood elevation.
- The hCG diet usually works to lose weight. If there is a problem with the diet, there may be a problem with the hCG. It may have been left out of the refrigerator, or have been inactive when they got it from the pharmacy. Patients may be cheating on the diet. They may be taking in fat.
- Weight loss is maintained when finished with the 3-6 week protocol, *if* the maintenance diet is followed. People maintain the weight loss for six months or a year or longer later. This is a benefit that cannot be claimed by most other weight-loss methods, particularly pharmaceuticals.
- It is cost-effective when considering the short amount of time that it takes.
- It is quick. Although the diet is very strict while you are on it, at the end you can resume your normal life again.
- Health improves.
    o Patients with type-2 diabetes improve.
    o Hypertension improves.
    o Those who have medical issues with being overweight can expect to improve those problems.

11. The Use of HCG is Controversial.

(1) CLINICAL STUDIES. Results are conflicting. Some studies show the hCG protocol to be effective, and others don't. More research is needed. [37 38 39 40 41 42 43 44 45]

Bad hCG batches may be the reason for the discrepancy in findings. One explanation for the conflicting data may be found in the stability of the hCG used in the studies. When looking at the studies that found no advantages to the hCG protocol, especially in the older studies, the stability of the hCG may be questioned.

Bad batches of hCG are not uncommon, even today, even from big reputable pharmacies. Another reason for the discrepancy in findings may be that many of these studies did not follow the dosing and diet protocol as outlined by Dr. Simeons.

(2) The Federal Trade Commission (FTC) in 1976 ordered Simeons Management Corporation, Simeons Weight Clinics foundation, Bariatrics Management Corporation, and HCG Weight Clinics Foundation to stop claiming that hCG-based programs were safe, effective, and/or approved by the FDA for weight control.

They required that patients who were receiving treatment be informed in writing: "These weight reduction treatments include the injection of hCG, a drug which has not been approved by the FDA as safe and effective in the treatment of obesity. There is no substantial evidence that hCG increases weight loss beyond that resulting from caloric restriction, that it causes a more "normal" distribution of fat, or that it decreases the hunger and discomfort associated with calorie-restricted diets."

(3) The FDA. In the early 70s, hCG was the most widespread obesity medication administered in the United States. Since 1975, the FDA has required labeling and advertising of hCG which states: "HCG has not been demonstrated to be effective adjunctive therapy in the treatment of obesity. There is no substantial evidence that it increases weight loss beyond that resulting from caloric restriction, that it causes a more attractive or normal distribution of fat, or that it decreases the hunger and discomfort associated with calorie-restricted diets."

The FDA has recently begun to crack down on internet sellers of hCG products. These products may soon become unavailable.

(4) HCG is not FDA-approved for weight loss. It is not

standard of care, meaning it is not prescribed for weight loss by a majority of physicians. As hCG is not FDA-approved for the treatment of obesity, a physician can only prescribe it for "off-label usage." This means that it is being used outside FDA indications. This is legal, as the FDA does not have the legal authority to regulate the practice of medicine. It is, however, illegal for the manufacturers to directly market a drug for uses other than FDA-approved indications. Thus you will not see a commercial for hCG and weight loss on TV.

A physician prescribing hCG must notify the patient that the proposed treatment is off-label use and have the patient sign a consent form for the off-label use. Your doctor is probably not covered by his malpractice carrier for this off-label use. This makes him/her liable for negligence or any complications of treatment and he or she may lose his/her license if any complications occur during the treatment.

If you are damaged by the treatment, you may need money for further care. Suing the doctor would be futile, as he/she would not be covered and would possibly be unable to compensate you for your damages.

12. Side Effects and Complications

SIDE EFFECTS AND COMPLICATIONS:

- Gout.
- Hair loss (no irreversible cases).
- Menstrual irregularities.[46]
- Gall bladder issues.[47] [48]
- Headache.[49]
- Loss of energy.
- Ovarian hyperstimulation syndrome.

Without physician supervision, obese patients will be at greater risk for heart attack, stroke, and other serious complications not usually associated with these therapies.

Contraindications:

If you have any of these conditions, you should not consider doing the hCG protocol:

- Pregnancy.
- Severe heart disease.
- Cancer.
- Polycystic ovarian syndrome.[50]
- Kidney disease.
- Seizures.
- Severe respiratory illnesses.

There is a potential for gout arthritis. Uric acid levels go higher with the hCG protocol.[51] You are living on ketones, because this is a starvation mode. These ketones compete with uric acid for excretion from the kidneys. If uric acids levels rise, or there is a history of gout arthritis, the doctor may want to prescribe anti-gout medications to keep the uric acid levels down, if that is a medically prudent thing to do for that patient.

Women who are cycling may have irregular bleeding as the hCG pushes the ovaries to make more hormones. These effects only last during the hCG injection period.

Those with type-2 diabetes who are on insulin and other meds should monitor blood sugar very carefully. The doctor supervising these patients may advise them to reduce their meds when starting the program with the calorie restriction. Otherwise, hypoglycemia may result. These patients require close medical supervision.

You may experience dangerous toxic reactions. The toxic poisons in our bodies are all fat-soluble. When you lose a pound of fat, those toxins are released into the blood. If not eliminated, they may redistribute, possibly to vulnerable sites like the brain or the kidneys.

There have been anecdotal reports of pancreatic dysfunction after doing the hCG protocol, especially in the elderly. If your pancreas is weakened, homeopathics may be helpful in restoring health to it and other organs that have been damaged by the toxicity.

If you feel ill on the hCG diet, that is the first warning that toxicity is being released into the bloodstream. A coffee enema will reduce the levels of toxins in the blood, and the loss of symptoms will be diagnostic or toxicity as well as therapeutic.

If you do have symptoms of toxicity, do not do this diet without careful attention to cleansing procedures. Even if you don't feel toxic symptoms, take this opportunity to detoxify and cleanse your body while you are losing weight. We all have PCBs, phthalates from plastics, insecticide residues, heavy metals, and other poisons that have been accumulating for a lifetime in our fat. So get them out. If you don't cleanse, the toxins that are released from the fat will be redistributed into the remaining fat and tissues again. Or you will get sick as your body throws them off with or without your help. It's more comfortable to take coffee enemas than to experience illness. Please read Secrets about Bioidentical Hormones, Chapter 27 and do the cleansing procedures described there.[52]

13. F.A.Q. About HCG

COULD I LOSE THE SAME AMOUNT OF WEIGHT on a very low calorie diet without hCG? Yes. But without the hCG you will experience loss of muscle, decreased vitality, increased fatigue, deranged hormones, and loss of energy.

What happens if I binge? It is a good idea to start the diet at a time when you are not planning to go on vacation for a while. Vacations make it tougher to stick with the plan. But there are probably going to be days when you binge. Do some cardio work to get your insulin levels to drop lower.

If I am not losing weight, should I stop taking Omega 3's? Omega 3's are very helpful, but if you aren't losing the weight while taking them, you can try dropping these and all other fats while on the protocol and add them back later.

I am an athlete in competition. Can I go on the hCG diet? Yes. But you would need to increase your calories. Try to stay with the protocol of protein, fruit, and veggies and stay away from the starchy carbs. You can still change your metabolism and get long-term weight loss. If you are working out a lot, you can still do the hCG diet, but you will need to add more calories.

I feel so great when I am on the hCG. Can I go ahead and keep taking it after the forty days are up? No. It is best to follow the protocol.

I have gained weight after being on the hCG diet. What should I do? Go back and see your doctor. Make sure you are staying away from the sweeteners and preservatives and artificial foods, and have him/her check your hormone status.

14.   Before Trying the HCG Protocol . . .

SO... HCG IS A CONTROVERSIAL WAY to lose unwanted fat. Physicians have strong biases both ways, but there are thousands and thousands of proponents of the hCG diet. Many people love the hCG protocol. Many patients who have followed the hCG treatment protocol report that they have lost weight, sleep better, are not as weak and irritable, and have shed inches in body circumference. These patients also report diminishment of other health concerns. The hCG protocol still remains a popular patient choice. Many physicians have successfully prescribed the protocol without patient complications and with great results.

Before trying hCG, first balance your hormones, correct your diet, exercise, sleep 8-9 hrs each night, and de-stress. Read Book One in the "Bioidentical Hormone" series, Secrets to Lose Fat and Keep It Off Forever! Balance Your Hormones: Insulin, Estrogen, Progesterone, Testosterone, Thyroid, Cortisol, and DHEA! Also read Book Five, Fat Loss Secrets that Really Work! Balance Your Hormones: Insulin, Estrogen, Progesterone, Testosterone, Thyroid, Cortisol, and DHEA! You may be able to lose the weight that you need to lose *without* using the hCG protocol.

Use the hCG protocol only under a doctor's supervision. We still don't have a complete understanding of hCG. More research is needed. If you decide to try it, do it under a physician's supervision.This protocol has been proven to be effective, but does have side effects and complications that may occur. Make sure you detoxify properly and adhere strictly to the guidelines outlined in the hCG protocol.

You will lose the fat and keep it off if you use this information! If you set your intention to lose the fat and keep it off, with the help of this book, you will succeed. Refer to the book often and the expanded information in Secrets about Bioidentical Hormones! [53] Good luck following the program!

INDEX

REFERENCES

[1] Dos Santos E, Dieudonné MN, Leneveu MC, Pecquery R, Serazin V, Giudicelli Y. In vitro effects of chorionic gonadotropin hormone on human adipose development. *J Endocrinol. 2007 Aug;194(2):313-25.*

[2] Norris W, Nevers T, Sharma S, Kalkunte S. Review: hCG, preeclampsia and regulatory T cells. *Placenta. 2011 Mar;32 Suppl 2:S182-5. Review.*

[3] Wan H, Coppens JM, van Helden-Meeuwsen CG, Leenen PJ, van Rooijen N, Khan NA, Kiekens RC, Benner R, Versnel MA. Chorionic gonadotropin alleviates thioglycollate-induced peritonitis by affecting macrophage function. *J Leukoc Biol. 2009 Aug;86(2):361-70.*

[4] Fleigelman R, Fried GH. Metabolic effects of human chorionic gonadotropin (HCG) in rats. *Proc Soc Exp Biol Med. 1970 Nov;135(2):317-9.*

[5] Vogt T, Belluscio D. Controversies in plastic surgery: suction-assisted lipectomy (SAL) and the hCG (human chorionic gonadotropin) protocol for obesity treatment. *Aesthetic Plast Surg. 1987;11(3):131-56. Review.*

[6] Efficacy and safety of highly purified urinary follicle-stimulating hormone with human chorionic gonadotropin for treating men with isolated hypogonadotropic hypogonadism. *European Metrodin HP Study Group. Fertil Steril. 1998 Aug;70(2):256-62.*

[7] Tsutsumi R, Fujimoto A, Osuga Y, Harada M, Takemura Y, Koizumi M, Yano T, Taketani Y. Successful pregnancy following low-dose hCG administration in addition to hMG in a patient with hypothalamic amenorrhea due to weight loss. *Gynecol Endocrinol. 2011 Nov 21.*

[8] Asher WL, Harper HW. Effect of human chorionic gonadotropin on weight loss, hunger, and feeling of well-being. *Am J Clin Nutr. 26: Feb 1973: 211-218.*

[9] Yaginuma T. Uptake of labeled human chorionic gonadotrophin in the brain of the adult female rat. *Acta Endocrinol (Copenh). 1972 Oct;71(2):245-54.*

[10] Vogt T, Belluscio D. Controversies in plastic surgery: suction-assisted lipectomy (SAL) and the hCG (human chorionic gonadotropin) protocol for obesity treatment. *Aesthetic Plast Surg. 1987;11(3):131-56. Review.*

[11] Simeons AT. The action of chorionic gonadotrophin in the obese. *Lancet. 1954 Nov 6;267(6845):946-7.*

[12] Simeons AT. Chorionic Gonadotropin in the treatment of obesity. *Am J Clin Nutr. 1964 Sep;15:188-90.*

[13] Vogt T, Belluscio D. Controversies in plastic surgery: suction-assisted lipectomy (SAL) and the hCG (human chorionic gonadotropin) protocol for obesity treatment. *Aesthetic Plast Surg. 1987;11(3):131-56.*

[14] Chan CC, Ng EH, Chan MM, Tang OS, Lau EY, Yeung WS, Ho PC. Bioavailability of hCG after intramuscular or subcutaneous injection in obese and non-obese women. *Hum Reprod. 2003 Nov;18(11):2294-7.*

[15] Toffle RC. "There they go again"--hCG and weight loss. *W V Med J. 2011 Jan-Feb;107(1):12-3.*

[16] Blackburn GL. Comparison of medically supervised and unsupervised approaches to weight loss and control. *Ann Intern Med. 1993 Oct 1;119(7 Pt 2):714-8. Review.*

[17] Wright, YL. *Fat Loss Secrets that Really Work--Balance Your Hormones: Insulin, Estrogen, Progesterone, Testosterone, Thyroid, Cortisol, and DHEA!* Lulu.com. 2011.

[18] http://www.worldhealth.net/pages/directory/ 888-997-0112

[19] http://www.acamnet.org/ 800-532-3688

[20] Santos JE, Thatcher WW, Pool L, Overton MW. Effect of human chorionic gonadotropin on luteal function and reproductive performance of high-producing lactating Holstein dairy cows. *J Anim Sci. 2001 Nov;79(11):2881-94.*

[21] Graham LH, Swanson WF, Brown JL. Chorionic gonadotropin administration in domestic cats causes an abnormal endocrine environment that disrupts oviductal embryo transport. *Theriogenology. 2000 Oct 15;54(7):1117-31.*

[22] Ishimaru T. Plasma estradiol concentrations and effect of HCG on plasma estradiol and testosterone in normal subjects and patients with endocrine disorders. *Endocrinol Jpn. 1975 Aug;22(4):287-96.*

[23] Wright YL. *Secrets about Bioidentical Hormones to Lose Fat and Prevent Cancer, Heart Disease, Menopause, and Andropause, by Optimizing Adrenals, Thyroid, Estrogen, Progesterone, Testosterone, and Growth Hormone!* Lulu.com. 2010.

[24] Wright YL. *Bioidentical Hormones Made Easy!* Lulu.com. 2011

[25] Wright YL. *Secrets about Bioidentical Hormones to Lose Fat and Prevent Cancer, Heart Disease, Menopause, and Andropause, by Optimizing Adrenals, Thyroid, Estrogen, Progesterone, Testosterone, and Growth Hormone!* Lulu.com. 2010. p 48.

[26] Wilson JH, Lamberts SW. The effect of triiodothyronine on weight loss and nitrogen balance of obese patients on a very-low-calorie liquid-formula diet. Int J Obes. 1981;5(3):279-82.

[27] Wright YL. *Secrets about Bioidentical Hormones to Lose Fat and Prevent Cancer, Heart Disease, Menopause, and Andropause, by Optimizing Adrenals, Thyroid, Estrogen, Progesterone, Testosterone, and Growth Hormone!* Lulu.com. 2010

[28] Wright YL.   *Secrets About Growth Hormone To Build Muscle Mass, Increase Bone Density, and Burn Body Fat!* Lulu.com, 2011.

[29] Mikirova NA, Casciari JJ, Hunninghake RE, Beezley MM. Effect of weight reduction on cardiovascular risk factors and CD34-positive cells in circulation. *Int J Med Sci. 2011;8(6):445-52.*

[30] Hugues JN. Comparative use of urinary and recombinant human chorionic gonadotropins in women. *Treat Endocrinol. 2004;3(6):371-9. Review.*

[31] Hermans P, Clumeck N, Picard O, van Vooren JP, Duriez P, Zucman D, Bryant JL, Gill P, Lunardi-Iskandar Y, Gallo RC. AIDS-related Kaposi's sarcoma patients with visceral manifestations. Response to human chorionic gonadotropin preparations. *J Hum Virol. 1998 Jan-Feb;1(2):82-9.*

[32] Efficacy and safety of highly purified urinary follicle-stimulating hormone with human chorionic gonadotropin for treating men with isolated hypogonadotropic hypogonadism. *European Metrodin HP Study Group. Fertil Steril. 1998 Aug;70(2):256-62.*

[33] Nargund G, Hutchison L, Scaramuzzi R, Campbell S. Low-dose HCG is useful in preventing OHSS in high-risk women without adversely affecting the outcome of IVF cycles. *Reprod Biomed Online. 2007 Jun;14(6):682-5.*

[34] Lopez D, Sekharam M, Coppola D, Carter WB. Purified human chorionic gonadotropin induces apoptosis in breast cancer. *Mol Cancer Ther. 2008 Sep;7(9):2837-44.*

[35] Bernstein L, Hanisch R, Sullivan-Halley J, Ross RK. Treatment with human chorionic gonadotropin and risk of breast cancer. *Cancer Epidemiol Biomarkers Prev. 1995 Jul-Aug;4(5):437-40.*

[36] Tennant FS, Hormone Treatments in Chronic and Intractable Pain. *Practical Pain Mgmt 2005; April, 57-67.*

[37] Rabe T, Richter S, Kiesel L, Runnebaum B. [Risk-benefit analysis of a hCG-500 kcal

reducing diet (cura romana) in females]. *Geburtshilfe Frauenheilkd. 1987 May;47(5):297-307.* German.

[38] Simeons AT. The action of chorionic gonadotrophin in the obese. *Lancet. 1954 Nov 6;267(6845):946-7.*

[39] Belluscio DO. Ripamonte L. and Wolanski M. "Utility of an oral presentation of hCG for the management of obesity: a double-blind study." *Copyright Dr. Daniel Belluscio 1994-1997.*

[40] Bosch B, Venter I, Stewart RI, Bertram SR. Human chorionic gonadotrophin and weight loss—a double-blind, placebo-controlled trial. *S Afr Med J. 1990 Feb 17; 77(4):185-9.*

[41] Shetty KR, Kalkhoff RK. Human chorionic gonadotropin (HCG) treatment of obesity. *Arch Intern Med. 1977 Feb;137(2):151-5.*

[42] Greenway FL, Bray GA. Human chorionic gonadotropin (HCG) in the treatment of obesity: a critical assessment of the Simeons method. *West J Med. 1977 Dec;127(6):461-3.*

[43] Stein MR, Julis RE, Peck CC, Hinshaw W, Sawicki JE, Deller JJ Jr. Ineffectiveness of human chorionic gonadotropin in weight reduction: a double-blind study. *Am J Clin Nutr. 1976 Sep;29(9):940-8.*

[44] Young RL, Fuchs RJ, Woltjen MJ. Chorionic gonadotropin in weight control. A double-blind crossover study. *JAMA. 1976 Nov 29;236(22):2495-7.*

[45] Lijesen GK, Theeuwen I, Assendelft WJ, Van Der Wal G. The effect of human chorionic gonadotropin (HCG) in the treatment of obesity by means of the Simeons therapy: a criteria-based meta-analysis. *Br J Clin Pharmacol. 1995 Sep;40(3):237-43.*

[46] Friedrich F, Kemeter P, Salzer H, Breitenecker G. Ovulation inhibition with human chorionic gonadotrophin. *Acta Endocrinol (Copenh). 1975 Feb;78(2):332-42.*

[47] Wadera S, Magid MS, McOmber M, Carpentieri D, Miloh T. Atypical presentation of Wilson disease. *Semin Liver Dis. 2011 Aug;31(3):319-26.*

[48] Kamrath RO, Plummer LJ, Sadur CN, Adler MA, Strader WJ, Young RL, Weinstein RL. Cholelithiasis in patients treated with a very-low-calorie diet. *Am J Clin Nutr. 1992 Jul;56(1 Suppl):255S-257S.*

[49] Rabe T, Richter S, Kiesel L, Zaloumis M, Runnebaum B. [Influence of human chorionic gonadotropin (hCG) in combination with a 500 calorie diet on clinical and laboratory parameters in premenopausal women with and without hormonal contraception]. *Aktuel Endokrinol Stoffwechsel. 1987 Jul;8(3):142-9.* German.

[50] Bruot BC. Hormone secretion by euthyroid and hypothyroid rat ovaries during the early stages of hCG-induced ovarian cyst development. *Proc Soc Exp Biol Med. 1987 Feb;184(2):206-10.*

[51] Arai K, Miura J, Ohno M, Yokoyama J, Ikeda Y. Comparison of clinical usefulness of very-low-calorie diet and supplemental low-calorie diet. *Am J Clin Nutr. 1992 Jul;56(1 Suppl):275S-276S.*

[52] Wright YL. *Secrets about Bioidentical Hormones to Lose Fat and Prevent Cancer, Heart Disease, Menopause, and Andropause, by Optimizing Adrenals, Thyroid, Estrogen, Progesterone, Testosterone, and Growth Hormone!* Lulu.com. 2010. p 66.

[53] Wright YL. *Secrets about Bioidentical Hormones to Lose Fat and Prevent Cancer, Heart Disease, Menopause, and Andropause, by Optimizing Adrenals, Thyroid, Estrogen, Progesterone, Testosterone, and Growth Hormone!* Lulu.com. 2010.

www.ingramcontent.com/pod-product-compliance
Lightning Source LLC
Chambersburg PA
CBHW031335290526
45784CB00014B/2757